MW00931976

THE ULTIMATE GUIDE TO DICLOFENAC

The Step by Step Guide Used to Relieve Pain,Swelling(Inflammation) and Joint Stiffness Caused by Arthritis Including Treatment of Osteoarthritis,Rheumatoid Arthritis and Ankylosing Spondylitis

ISBN 978-1-4583-0976-1

Marik Bonder

TABLE OF CONTENT

CHAPTER 1

INTRODUCTION

Diclofenac is a medication that is used to treat swelling (inflammation) and pain in the body.

Among its many applications are the treatment of aches and pains, as well as issues with joints, muscles, and bones, among others. These are some examples:

Osteoarthritis and rheumatoid arthritis are the two most common kinds of the disease.

Muscle and ligament sprains and strains are common injuries.

back aches and pains

toothache

migraine

gout

Ankylosing spondylitis (also known as degenerative disc disease) is an inflammation of the spine and other regions of the body.

Diclofenac is available in a variety of forms, including pills and capsules, including slow-release tablets and capsules, as well as suppositories. These are only accessible with a doctor's prescription.

Anti-inflammatory medications such as diclofenac gel and plasters for joint discomfort are available for purchase from pharmacies.

It may also be administered intravenously or topically via the eyes. These are often only administered in a hospital setting.

Actinic keratoses are treated with a diclofenac gel that has a high concentration of diclofenac (3 percent diclofenac) (dry, scaly patches of skin caused by sun damage). This therapy is normally initiated after an evaluation by a dermatologist and is not discussed in this article.

CHAPTER 2

The most important information

To manage your symptoms, it is preferable to take the lowest possible dosage of diclofenac for the shortest amount of time.

It is recommended that you take diclofenac pills or capsules with a meal, snack, or immediately after eating.

Stomach ache, feeling or being ill, and rashes are all common adverse effects of this medication.

When you have pain in a specific location of your body, you may use Diclofenac gel and plasters twice a day to relieve it.

Who is permitted to use diclofenac and who is not

The majority of individuals are able to take diclofenac.

Diclofenac may be administered to children for the treatment of joint pain. Diclofenac pills, capsules, and suppositories are appropriate for use in children 6 months and older, but not in infants.

Diclofenac gel is appropriate for use in children aged 14 and older. Diclofenac plasters and patches are appropriate for use by adolescents and young adults aged 16 and above.

Some individuals are unable to use Diclofenac because of a medical condition. In order to ensure that it is safe for you, notify your doctor or pharmacist if you have any of the following conditions:

Have you ever had an adverse response to diclofenac or any other medications?

allergy to aspirin or other nonsteroidal anti inflammatory drugs (NSAIDs) such as ibuprofen or naproxetine

Has anybody in your family ever had adverse effects from using NSAIDs, such as wheezing or other indications of asthma, a runny nose, swelling of the skin (angioedema), or an allergic reaction to the medication?

Has anybody in your family ever had stomach ulcers, bleeding in the stomach or intestines, or a hole in the stomach?

have hypertension (high blood pressure) (hypertension)

you suffer from heart failure, severe liver illness, or renal damage

If you've been diagnosed with Crohn's disease or ulcerative colitis, you'll need to see your doctor.

afflicted with lupus

have a problem with blood clotting.

are pregnant, intending to get pregnant, or
are nursing a child

CHAPTER 3

HOW TO TAKE DICLOFENAC

How and when should diclofenac be taken or used

Keep in mind to always follow the advise of a pharmacist or doctor, as well as the directions included with your medication.

Dosage

You'll often take diclofenac pills, capsules, or suppositories 2 to 3 times each day, depending on your condition.

In most cases, the recommended daily amount is 75mg to 150mg, depending on what your doctor recommends for you.

Follow your doctor's instructions on the number of pills to take and how many times to take them each day.

If your doctor prescribes diclofenac for your kid, they will calculate the appropriate dosage for your child based on the weight of your child.

If you suffer from chronic pain, your doctor may prescribe slow-release diclofenac pills or capsules to you. In most cases, you'll take them once a day in the evening or twice a day in the morning. If you're taking slow-release diclofenac twice a day, you should wait 10 to 12 hours between doses to avoid stomach upset.

What to do while using pills and capsules

Take diclofenac pills or capsules with a glass of milk to get the most benefit. If you have to take them with water, wait until after a meal or snack before taking them. If you take them with milk or food, you will be less likely to have an upset or irritated stomach from them.

Do not crush, shatter, or chew them; instead, swallow them whole.

When and how should you utilize suppositories

Suppositories are medications that are inserted softly into the anus of the patient (bottom)

If you need to, use the restroom before the meeting.

Hands should be washed before and after taking the medication. Clean the region around your anus with gentle soap and water, then rinse and pat dry.

Remove the suppository from its packaging.

Inject the suppository into your anus by gently pushing it in with the pointed end first. It has to be inserted around 3 cm into the hole (1 inch).

For about 15 minutes, sit or lay motionless. The suppository will dissolve as it enters your stomach. This is quite normal.

Diclofenac gel is a topical analgesic.

Dosage

Depending on how powerful the gel is, you'll often apply it 2 to 4 times each day, on average. More information may be found on the box, or you can chat with your pharmacist.

If you're going to use the gel twice a day, use it once in the morning and once in the evening to your face and neck. If you're using it three or four times a day, you should wait at least four hours between applications.

The quantity of gel you will use will be determined by the size of the region you want to treat. Most of the time, you'll utilize a quantity that's roughly the size of a 1 cent or 2 penny piece (2 to 4 grams).

It is important to note that the maximum dosage of diclofenac gel is 20 mg.

It is not recommended to use diclofenac gel more than four times in a 24-hour period.

How to make use of the gel

To get a little quantity of gel, gently squeeze the tube, or push firmly and evenly on the nozzle of the dispenser, as appropriate.

Using your fingers, gently massage the gel into the sore or swollen region. It is possible that it will feel chilly on your skin. After that, wash your hands well.

Plasters and patches containing diclofenac

Dosage

Only one sore location should be treated at a time. In any 24-hour period, do not use more than 2 medicated plasters or patches containing medication.

Plasters and patches: how to apply them

Apply a medicinal plaster or patch to the sore region twice a day, once in the morning and once in the evening, until the pain subsides completely. You must first remove the previous patch before applying the new one.

Apply mild pressure to the skin with the palm of your hand until it is thoroughly adhered to the surface.

When removing a plaster or patch, it is advisable to wet the area first with some water before doing so. Once the adhesive has been removed, wash the afflicted area and gently massage it in circular motions to remove any remaining glue.

What happens if I don't remember to take it?

You should take diclofenac as soon as you recall if you have forgotten to do so, unless it is almost time for your next dosage. The missed dosage should be skipped and the next one should be taken at the regular time.

Never take a double dosage in order to make up for a missed medication.

If you are prone to forgetting dosages, setting an alarm to remind you may be beneficial. You might also consult with your pharmacist for suggestions on alternative strategies to help you remember to take your medication.

What happens if I consume too much?

If you take more diclofenac pills, capsules, or suppositories than your doctor has advised, you might be in danger. It has the potential to create adverse effects such as:

a pain in the stomach

being unwell or having the sensation of being sick (vomiting) diarrhoea

If you have black feces or blood in your
vomit, this is a symptom that your stomach
is bleeding.

headaches

drowsiness

a ringing sensation in your ears (tinnitus)

And what happens if I use an excessive
number of plasters, patches, or gel?

If you use an excessive number of plasters
or patches, or an excessive amount of gel,

it is doubtful that you would suffer any consequences. However, if you use too much and have any negative effects, contact your doctor immediately.

Taking diclofenac in conjunction with other pain relievers

If you take diclofenac with paracetamol or codeine, you will be OK.

Do not use diclofenac with other pain relievers, such as aspirin, ibuprofen, or naproxen, without first seeing your physician.

Non-steroidal anti-inflammatory drugs (NSAIDs) include diclofenac, aspirin, ibuprofen, and naproxen, which are all members of the same class of medications (NSAIDs). Taking diclofenac alongside other nonsteroidal anti-inflammatory drugs (NSAIDs) may increase your risk of experiencing adverse effects such as stomach discomfort.

NSAIDs are also included in over-the-counter medications, such as cough and cold treatments, that may be purchased from pharmacies.

Important

Before taking any other medications with diclofenac, read the label to determine whether they include ibuprofen, aspirin, or other nonsteroidal anti-inflammatory drugs (NSAIDs).

CHAPTER 4

Adverse consequences

Diclofenac, like other medications, may produce adverse effects, but not everyone experiences them.

Consequences that are common

More than 1 in every 100 persons experience one or more of the common adverse effects of diclofenac pills, capsules, or suppositories.

If any of the following adverse effects annoy you or do not go away, see your doctor or pharmacist:

I'm feeling ill (nausea)

having diarrhea or getting ill (vomiting)

experiencing dizziness or vertigo

headaches

stomach soreness, wind, or a lack of
appetite are all possible symptoms.

a minor rash

When you use diclofenac gel or plasters,
you are less likely to have negative effects.
This is due to the fact that less medication
enters your body. However, you may still

have the same negative effects, particularly if you apply a big amount of product to a broad region of skin.

The use of diclofenac gel or plasters might have an adverse effect on your skin.

sunlight than the ordinary human being is more sensitive to

develop a rash on the skin where the gel or plaster was put

irritable or dehydrated (eczema)

irritated or inflamed (dermatitis)

Side effects that are potentially life-threatening

These major adverse effects are very uncommon, occurring in fewer than one person in every 1,000.

Call your doctor immediately if you experience any of the following:

If you have blood in your vomit or black feces, this might indicate that you have bleeding in your stomach or gut.

An ulcer or inflammation in your stomach or gut may manifest itself as severe indigestion, heartburn, or stomach discomfort, as well as vomiting or diarrhoea, amongst other symptoms.

Although it may be less noticeable on dark or black skin, the whites of your eyes or the skin around your mouth may become yellow. This might be an indication of liver troubles.

If you have a raised, itchy rash, or if your skin is swollen or puffy, you may be suffering from hives (urticaria) or oedema (swelling)

If you are experiencing shortness of breath, fatigue, or swelling in your legs or ankles, you may be suffering from heart failure.

How to deal with the adverse effects of diclofenac sodium

What should be done in this situation:

Diclofenac should be taken with or after a meal or snack if you are feeling unwell (nausea). It may also be beneficial to refrain from consuming fatty or spicy foods.

If you are feeling unwell (vomiting) or have diarrhea, drink lots of water or other fluids. If you're feeling under the weather, consider taking tiny, regular sips of water. If you notice indications of dehydration, such as urinating less often than normal or having black, foul-smelling urine, see a pharmacist right once. In the event that you are unwell or have diarrhea for more than 3 days, see a doctor. Do not take any additional medications without first consulting with a pharmacist or a doctor.

dizzy or unstable - If you are experiencing dizziness or vertigo, stop what you are doing and rest or lay down until you feel better. If you're feeling dizzy or lightheaded, avoid driving or cycling, as well as using tools or equipment. As your body becomes used to diclofenac, these side effects should gradually go away.

If you have a headache, make sure you get enough of rest and drink lots of water. Don't overindulge in alcoholic beverages. Inquire with your pharmacist for a recommendation on an alternate pain reliever. In most cases, headaches should subside within the first week of using diclofenac. If they linger more than a week or become severe, you should see your doctor.

stomach soreness, wind, or lack of appetite - avoid items that produce wind, such as fried meals (like peas, lentils, beans and onions). Eat smaller meals more often, chew and drink slowly, and engage in regular physical activity.

Skin irritation or dryness that is itchy or inflamed is caused by a slight rash. Apply emollient lotion or ointment to the afflicted region to moisturise, soothe and hydrate the skin. If the condition does not improve after a week or if you are concerned, see a pharmacist or a doctor.

Because your skin is more susceptible to sunlight, avoid direct sunlight and wear a high-factor sunscreen (SPF 15 or above) even on overcast days. Use of a sunlamp or sunbed is strictly prohibited.

CHAPTER 5

Pregnancy and nursing are important considerations.

In most cases, diclofenac is not suggested during pregnancy.

This is due to the possibility that diclofenac may create difficulties for your unborn child. It may, for example, have an effect on your baby's circulation and lead you to have too little amniotic fluid around your kid in the womb, both of which are harmful.

Your doctor will only recommend that you take diclofenac while you are pregnant if the dangers of not taking the medication exceed the benefits of doing so.

There may be other therapies that are less harmful to you. In general, paracetamol is the most effective pain reliever to use when pregnant.

Taking diclofenac during nursing is not recommended.

You may take diclofenac when you are nursing your child. There are just trace quantities that get into breast milk, and they are unlikely to produce any adverse consequences in your infant. It has been used successfully by many nursing women without any issues.

Consult your midwife, health visitor, pharmacist, or doctor immediately if you observe that your baby is not eating as well as normal, or if you have any other concerns about your baby's well-being.

Advice that is not time sensitive:

attempting to get pregnant

pregnant

breastfeeding

Continue reading this leaflet on diclofenac on the Best Use of Medicines in Pregnancy (BUMPs) website for further information on how this medication might impact you and your baby.

9. Precautions while using other medications

Some medications have been shown to have an effect on the way diclofenac works. You should tell your doctor if you're taking any of the accompanying:

Aspirin and ibuprofen, among other anti-inflammatory medications, are prescribed.

Antibiotics such as ciprofloxacin, levofloxacin, moxifloxacin, nalidixic acid, norfloxacin, and ofloxacin are examples of antimicrobial agents.

Anticoagulants (sometimes known as "blood thinners"), such as warfarin, are used to prevent blood clots.

Medicines for cardiac disorders, such as digoxin, and medications for excessive blood pressure are examples of such medications.

Colestipol and cholestyramine, two cholesterol-lowering medications, are examples.

phenytoin, for example, is a medication used to treat seizures.

Immunosuppressants, such as ciclosporin and tacrolimus, are medications that work by suppressing the activity of your immune system.

Antidepressants that are selective serotonin reuptake inhibitors (SSRIs), such as citalopram or sertraline, are prescribed.

Steroid medications, such as hydrocortisone or prednisolone, are used to treat inflammation.

Diuretics, such as furosemide and bumetanide, are medications that cause you to pee more.

Lithium is a medication that is used to treat mental health issues.

Methotrexate is a medication that is used to treat certain inflammatory illnesses and malignancies.

Mifepristone is a medication that is used to terminate a pregnancy (abortion)

Zidovudine is a medication that is used to treat HIV.

Combining diclofenac with herbal treatments or nutritional supplements is not recommended.

It is not feasible to determine whether or not supplementary medications or herbal therapies are safe to use in conjunction with diclofenac in this situation.

They are not subjected to the same rigorous testing as prescription medications or over-the-counter medications. They are not often evaluated for the interaction that they may have with other medications.

THE END

Made in the USA
Monee, IL
28 June 2024